DIY Placenta Encapsulation: A Step-By-Step Guide

By Katie DiBenedetto

Copyright 2014, by Katie DiBenedetto {2 Doulas on a Mission}

All rights reserved. No part of this book may be reproduced or transmitted in any form or by any means, electronic or mechanical, including photocopying and recording, or by any information storage or retrieval system, without permission in writing from the publisher. For requests or permission, please contact 2 Doulas on a Mission.

All photos are property of 2 Doulas on a Mission. For requests or permission, please contact 2 Doulas on a Mission.

Warning/Disclaimer: this guide is intended for personal use only, meaning for those intending to prepare their own personal placenta in their own home with their own equipment and supplies. This is not a guide for preparing ANYONE ELSES PLACENTA BUT YOUR OWN. Preparing other peoples placentas introduces a whole host of other considerations pertaining to personal health and safety that are not covered in this guide.

All placenta handling and preparation is done at your own risk. Katie DiBenedetto and 2 Doulas on a Mission shall have neither liability nor responsibility to any person or entity regarding any alleged loss, damage or injury as a result of the information presented in this work.

Acknowledgements

Special thanks to Nancy, who trusted me with her placenta (my first one!) even though I didn't know what I was doing. To Kewal, who instructed me how to prepare Nancy's placenta. To Danielle, my partner in learning for those first few placentas. And to Shell Walker, who started the Placenta Liberation Front (just one of many of her brilliant ventures), which provides an incredibly thorough and completely complimentary training on placenta prep, the only requirement being that you obtain all of the necessary supplies for professionalism and safety, that you go forward and teach other people, and provide your first few placenta preparations for free. I have learned so much from Shell and am grateful that my path has crossed hers in this life.

Table of Contents

Preface

Placenta Benefits

Safety & Sanitation

Supplies List + Where to Buy

Placenta Capsules, "Raw" Method

Placenta Capsules, "TCM" Method

Dosage & Storage

Resources

Preface

I wrote this guide for women. For women who perhaps aren't surrounded by other womenfolk who are full of knowledge and wisdom. For women who are curious. For women who want to know. For women knowing they want to do something with their placenta, but aren't quite sure what to do. For women who want somewhere to start, some steps to follow, some photos to help them along. I hope you find what you are looking for here ☺

Every time I see a posting or hear of a woman who's sad that she can't find an encapsulationist in her area, or bummed that encapsulation is out of her budget I think – I hope this mama knows she can do it herself! Or have her partner/friend/sister help her. Have we gotten so far away from our inner knowing and wisdom that we do not believe we are capable of preparing for our own consumption our own organ that we just spent 9 months growing inside of our own bodies? This is just silly.

Placenta crafting is not and should not be a "secret" that is guarded by "professionals". It is an act of love and gratitude that takes nothing more than a pair of capable hands and a few simple tools.

I am honored anytime a woman trusts me with the preparation of her placenta. Though I am delighted that it is one of the ways I sustain myself, I would never hesitate to empower a woman with the same knowledge and skills that I learned from my women friends and teachers. The wisdom that I hope you will pass on to your daughters, your friends and your sisters.

From my heart to yours,

Katie

Feel free to contact me with any questions that come up!
Katie@2doulasonamission.com

Placenta Benefits

The benefits of consuming your placenta are endless! Did you know that, other than camels, humans are the only mammal that doesn't consume their placenta? First and foremost, the placenta is an organ, so it is chock full of iron & other nutrients. On top of that – your placenta is full of hormones, which help balance your system after birth.

- Contains your own natural hormones

- Is perfectly made by you, for you

- Balances your system & replenishes depleted iron

- Gives you more energy & lessens postpartum bleeding

- Has been shown to increase milk production

- Helps you to have a happier postpartum period by equalizing the quickly reduced hormonal state of your physical body

- Helps to hasten the return of your uterus to its pre-pregnancy state through the oxytocin contained in your placenta.

- Helpful during your monthly cycle, menopause, for general mood swings, periods of major life transition, etc. if properly stored for later use.

- Visit our website – 2doulasonamission.com - for other articles & info about placentas.

Safety & Sanitation

As stated in the opening disclaimer (which is a bit harsh but, you know, necessary in this big world) this guide is not intended for use by anyone other than the individual woman (and her trusted family and friends) preparing her own placenta in her own home with her own equipment. May I reiterate that this is not at all the appropriate way to learn about placenta preparation if you are intending to have a placenta business and prepare the placentas of women that you don't know. If you are inspired to offer it as a service to your community – thank you! We need more women like you! Just please make sure you are properly trained and learn the necessary safety procedures with regards to sanitation, blood borne pathogens, etc.

As I'm sure you know, placentas are messy. It would be wise to clear yourself an area – a countertop, a table, somewhere that will minimize blood drips and splatters, simply for easier clean up. Make sure your area is large enough that you can have all of your supplies near you so you're not walking back and forth or scattered.

When you work with your placenta, be sure you are present and inspired. Put on your favorite music. Take a moment to thank your placenta and recognize what an amazing gift it gave to you and your baby. Try to keep your mind clear and your thoughts positive so as not to infuse your placenta with anything other than peaceful, joyful intentions and energy.

Supplies List + Where to Buy

Please note – this is not a list of everything you need to go out and buy. Some supplies are optional, some overlap, and some you only need for a specific method. This list is simply a reference guide for definitions of different supplies, where to get them, and what not to use. A simplified, supply list is listed with each method of encapsulation. Please make sure you read over this descriptive supplies list, decide what encapsulation method you want to use, and read through the instructions before you decide which supplies to get.

Scissors or a knife: I use stainless steel scissors that come completely apart. You can find these in the kitchen section of most stores. They're easy to clean and easily cut through the placenta. You could also use a knife – make sure it is very sharp. I would recommend partially freezing the placenta so that it is more solid and easier to slice with a knife.

Gloves – optional. Non-latex disposable gloves are best – the kind a doctor or nurse would use when doing an exam. I buy mine at Costco. Do not use plastic food prep gloves.

"Tray" – could be a cookie sheet, a tray, a cutting board or any other flat surface to place the placenta on while you're cutting it up. If you are using the raw method, it's helpful if your tray has a lip to aid in catching drips and keeping the blood contained. With the TCM Method you will have drained the placenta of blood so having a lip on your tray is not necessary.

Food dehydrator or oven. I use an Excalibur food dehydrator with 4 trays. It is solid and built to last – they often have sales and free shipping on their website. There is only one main difference with food dehydrators – the round dehydrators have the fan on top so they do not dry as effectively as square dehydrators, which have their fan at the back equally blowing on all of the trays. A round dehydrator is perfectly adequate, just know that it may take a bit longer and you may need to flip your pieces half way through. Round dehydrators are also much cheaper and easy to find on Craig's List. Make sure the dehydrator has an adjustable temperature setting so you can set it appropriately. You can also use your oven set at the lowest temperature if that is your only option. In my experience, it's worth picking up a used dehydrator on Craig's List versus using your oven. Even at the lowest setting, it will still be much hotter than a dehydrator, you'll have to flip all of your pieces part way through, and your oven will be on for a long time. However, if you don't mind all of that and you're not concerned with temperature or truly keeping the placenta "raw", then an oven is perfectly adequate – it's up to you. For simplicity, I'll instruct as if you're using a dehydrator.

Parchment paper (do not use wax paper!) This is optional, and is to line your dehydrator trays to make for easier clean up.

"Grinder" – you can use a coffee grinder, blender, food processor, mortar & pestle – whatever you want to use to turn your dried placenta strips into powder. In my experience, a coffee grinder or an electric nut and spice grinder gives you a perfect fine powder and is very quick and easy.

"Capsule Maker" This is optional, but makes for quicker capsule making. May not be worth it though if you don't think you're ever going to use your capsule maker again. You can just scoop and cap by hand. You can pick up one on Amazon, or locally at a vitamin store or herb shop. I use one made by the Capsule Connection.

Empty capsules – make sure your capsules are the same size as your capsule maker, if you're using one. Whole Foods (and some vitamin stores) sell empty capsules in the vitamin department. You can order them in bulk online as well. If you are vegetarian or vegan, make sure you look at the ingredients and get capsules made from vegetable cellulose, versus gelatin. The average placenta makes about 200 capsules.

A jar to store your finished capsules in. Make sure it's clean and dry. 200 capsules will fill up an 8 ounce jar.

Pot, steamer and lid – do not use a butterfly style steamer – this is nearly impossible to clean and the placenta will stick to it. A large colander type steamer or mesh basket steamer is best.

Placenta Capsules, "Raw" Method

The "raw" method of placenta encapsulation follows the ideas of the raw food principle that heat above 118 degrees degrades food and destroys essential nutrients, enzymes, etc. Using this method, the placenta is dehydrated at 115 degrees and is argued to have more hormones present and be more nutritionally dense. It is a very personal decision whether to use the raw method or the TCM style of placenta preparation. You can also do both! Prepare half of your placenta TCM style and half using the raw method. One is neither "right" nor "wrong", and no one besides the mother is to say what style of preparation is best for her.

Supplies

- Scissors
- 2 Trays
- Food dehydrator
- Grinder
- Empty capsules
- A jar

Optional

- Gloves
- Parchment paper
- Capsule Maker

Instructions

- Clear your area – remember, placentas are messy once you start cutting them up. Make sure you give yourself a good radius.
- Take out your dehydrator trays and lay them out in a single layer next to where you will be cutting up the placenta.
- If using parchment paper, line your dehydrator trays now
- Place your placenta on your first tray and cut off the membranes and the umbilical cord, if you haven't already. Save for later to preserve if you desire. (specific instructions in Volume 2)

- Cut the placenta into strips and pieces as if you were making beef jerky.
- Place the pieces in a single layer on your dehydrator trays

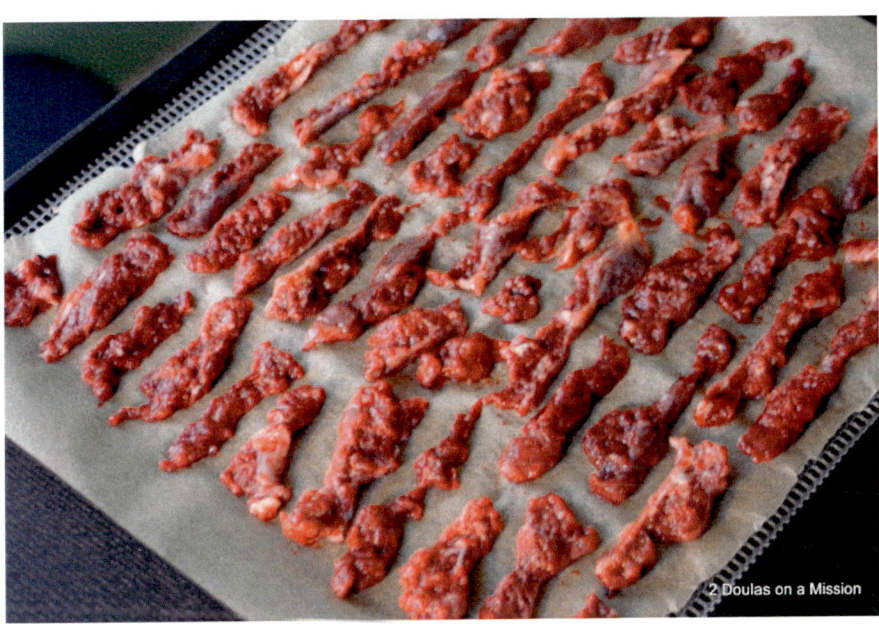

{raw placenta pieces ready to go on parchment paper lined dehydrator trays}

- Place the trays inside the dehydrator and set the temperature at 115 degrees. Typical drying time is 24-36 hours, sometimes longer, depending on how large/thick the placenta pieces are and what type of dehydrator you are using.
- If you don't have a dehydrator and are not concerned about temperature - you can lay the pieces of placenta out on a cookie sheet, lined with parchment paper if you desire, and dehydrate at the lowest temperature setting in your oven. Check pieces every couple of hours.

- To determine if your placenta is done: remove several different pieces from the dehydrator to test. They should all snap in half with absolutely no moisture present.

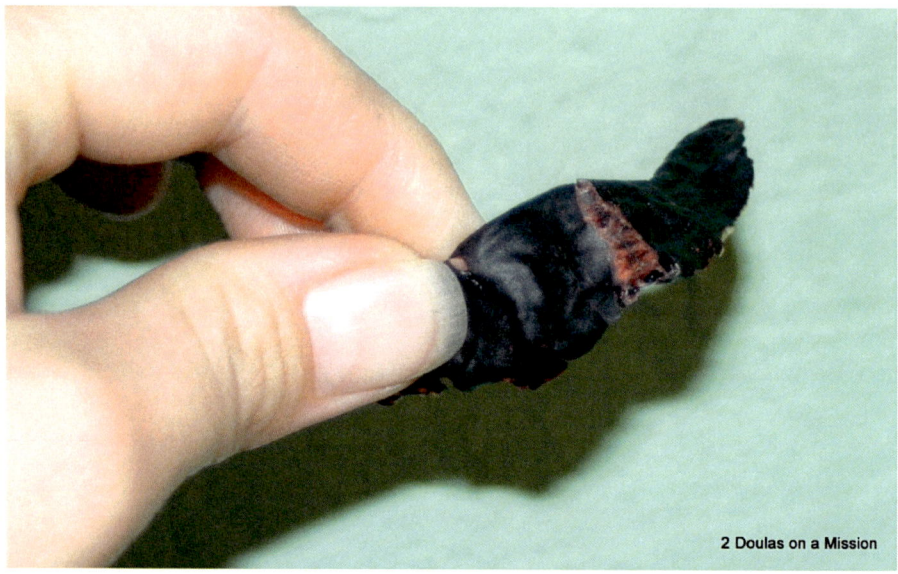

{example of a piece of placenta that is NOT fully dehydrated. It does not snap in half and it is still bright red and filled with moisture on the inside.}

- Once your pieces are dry, put them into your grinder. If you're using a coffee grinder it may take several rounds to get all of the pieces.
- Dump your powder onto your second tray

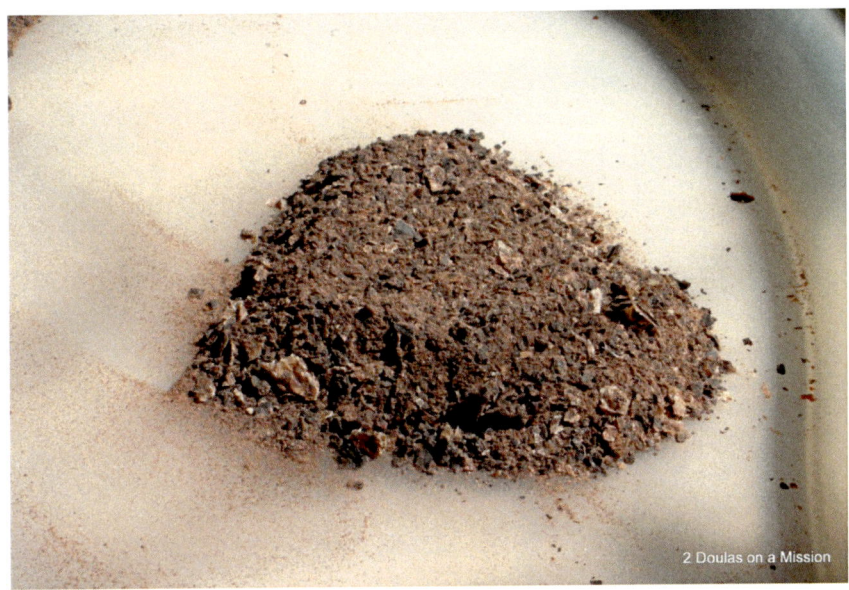

{dehydrated, ground placenta powder}

- Load capsule maker with the first round of empty capsules
- Use the spreader card to scoop the powder into the capsule maker

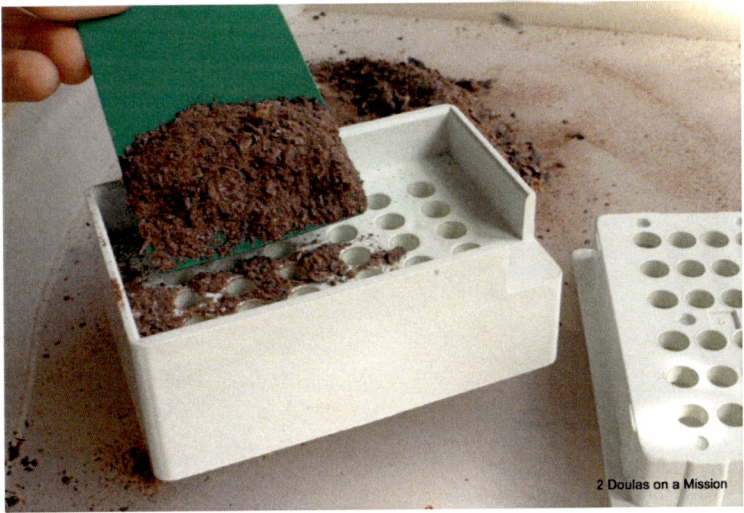

{scooping powder into the empty capsules with the spreader card}

- Use the tamper to tamp down once

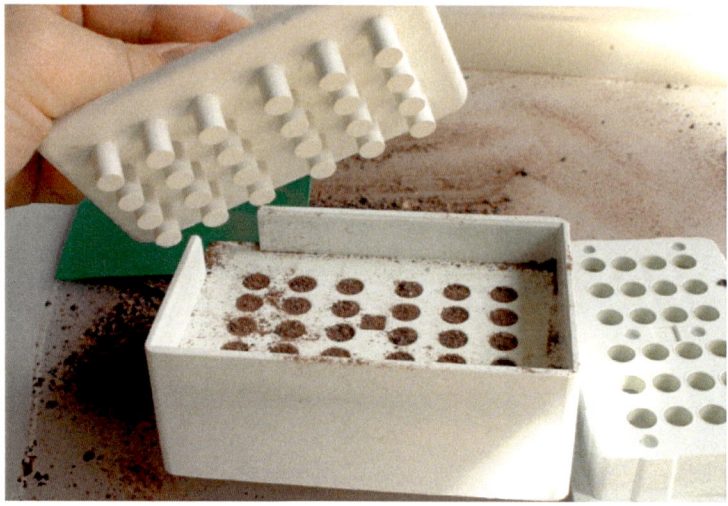

{using the tamper}

- Use spreader card to scoop more powder into the capsules
- Use spreader card to smooth things out & remove excess powder

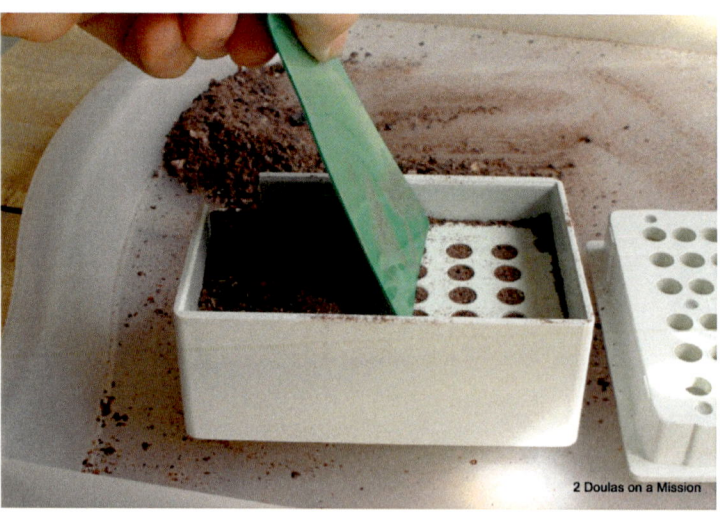

{using the spreader card to smooth out the placenta powder|

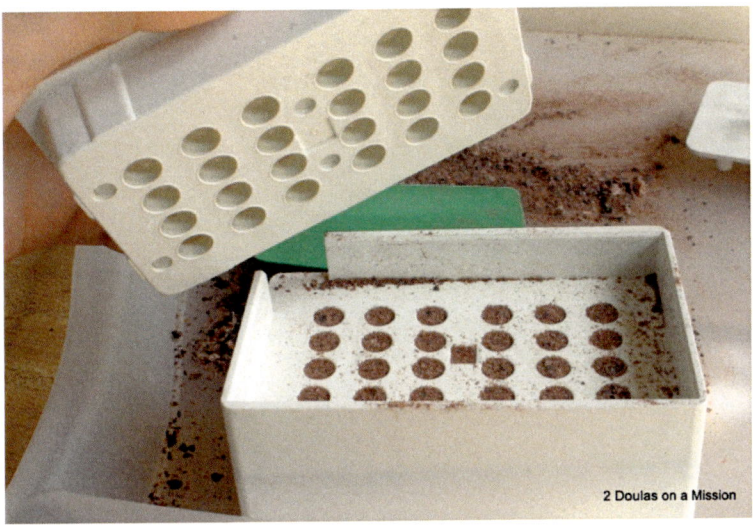

{matching up the top and bottom half}

- Push the top part and the bottom part of the capsule maker together and voila – sealed capsules
- Repeat until you have used all of your placenta powder

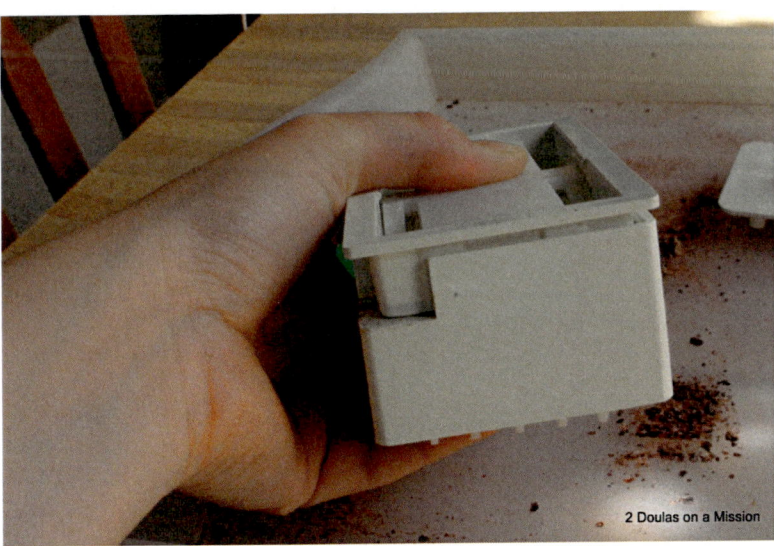

{pushing the top and bottom parts of the capsule maker together to seal the capsules}

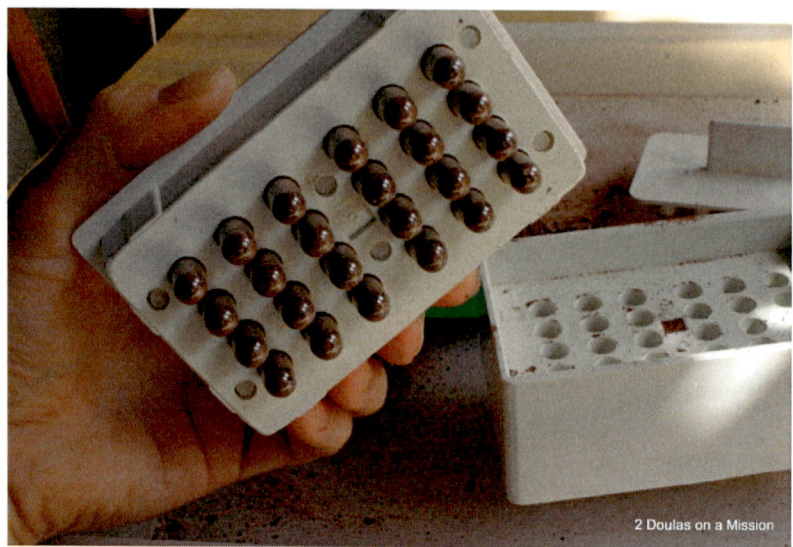

{Connected capsules!}

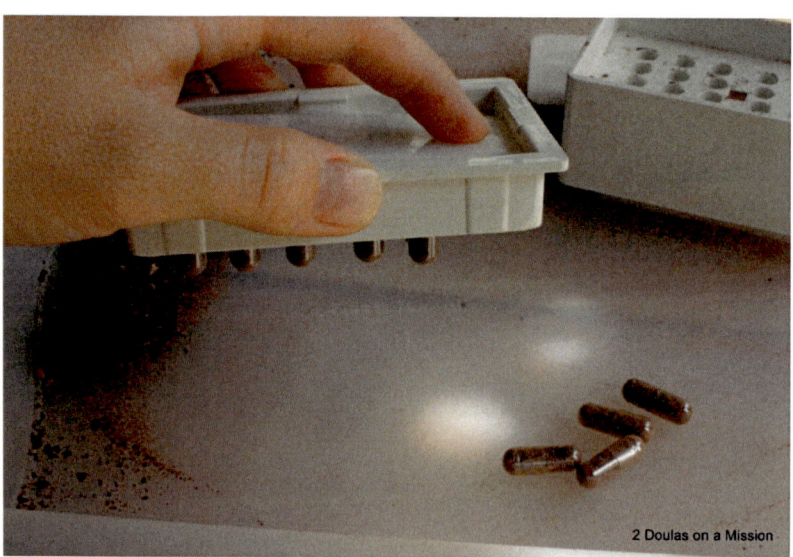

{pushing down on the top half to release the capsules}

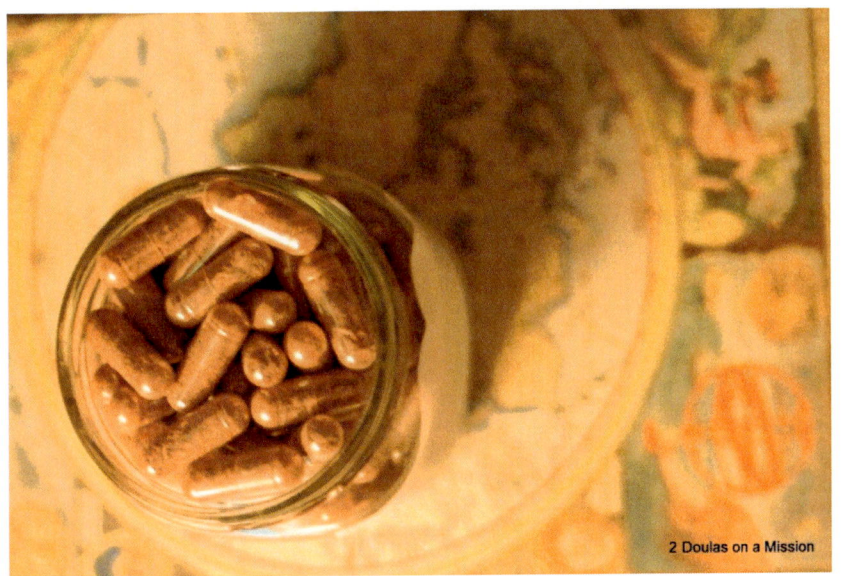

{finished capsules}

Placenta Capsules, "TCM" Method

TCM stands for Traditional Chinese Medicine. In Chinese medicine, it is believed that the process of birth leaves an empty open space full of lots of "yin" or "cold" energy. Therefore it is believed best to introduce only warming food, drink and supplements to a woman in the immediate postpartum period. The process of TCM placenta prep involves steaming the placenta with ginger, lime and jalapeno – introducing lots of warming energy back into the mother's body. It is a very personal decision whether to use the raw method or the TCM style of placenta preparation. You can also do both! Prepare half of your placenta TCM style and half using the raw method. One is neither "right" nor "wrong", and no one besides the mother is to say what style of preparation is best for her.

Supplies

- A strait pin
- Pot, steamer and lid
- 1" pieces of fresh ginger and jalapeno + several wedges of lime
- Scissors or a knife
- 2 Trays
- Food dehydrator
- Grinder
- Empty capsules
- A jar

Optional

- Capsule Maker
- Gloves
- Parchment paper

Instructions

- Clear out and sanitize the inside of your kitchen sink
- Put an inch or two of water in the pot for your steamer, along with you diced pieces of ginger & jalapeno and your lime wedges

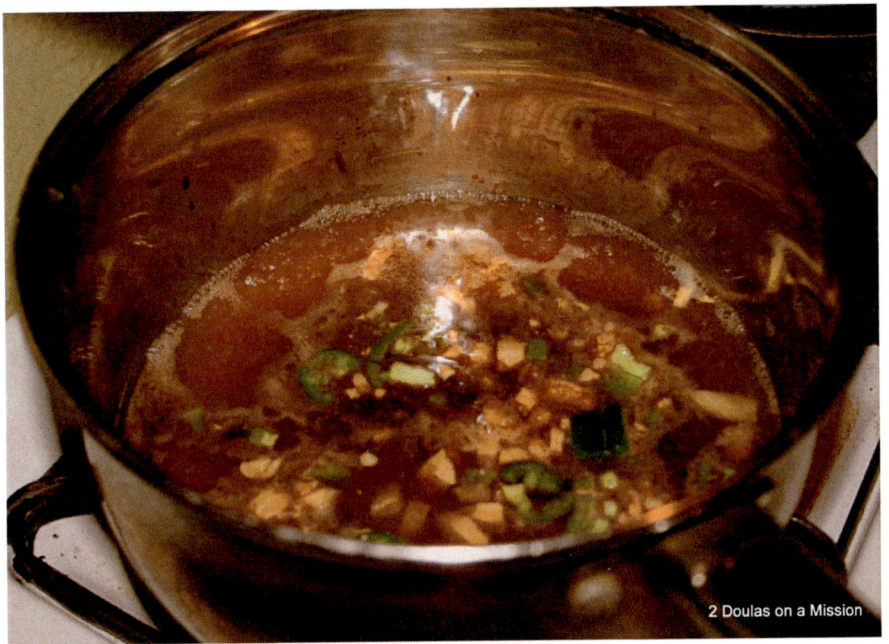

{Steamer pot ready with water, diced ginger and jalapeno and lime}

- Cut off the membranes and the umbilical cord, if you haven't already. Save for later to preserve if you desire (specific instructions in volume 2)
- Place the placenta in the sink with the faucet running slowly on it
- Begin massaging and rinsing the blood off of the placenta
- After a few minutes of massage, begin poking holes in various veins of the placenta and massage the blood out of the veins
- Once the placenta is adequately drained and rinsed (just do the best you can), place it in your steamer on your stove top and turn it on

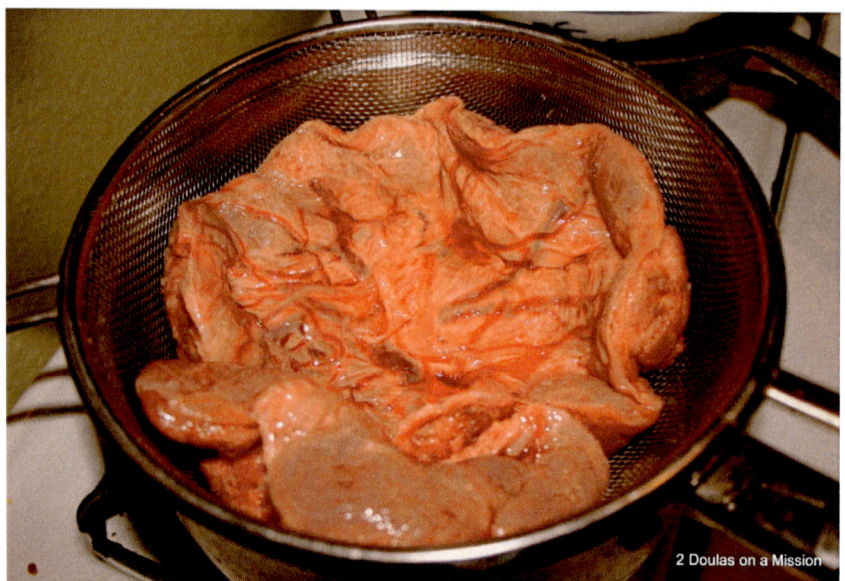

{rinsed placenta, read to be steamed}

- Steam for 20 minutes on each side

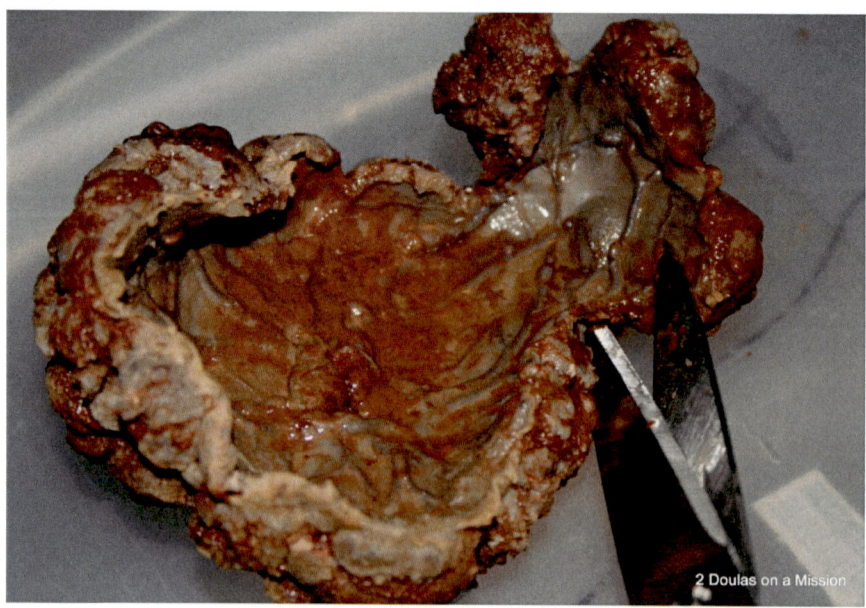

{Freshly steamed placenta, read to be sliced and dehydrated}

- Remove the placenta from the steamer and place it on your cutting board
- Once it's cool enough to handle, cut the placenta into strips as if you were making beef jerky.

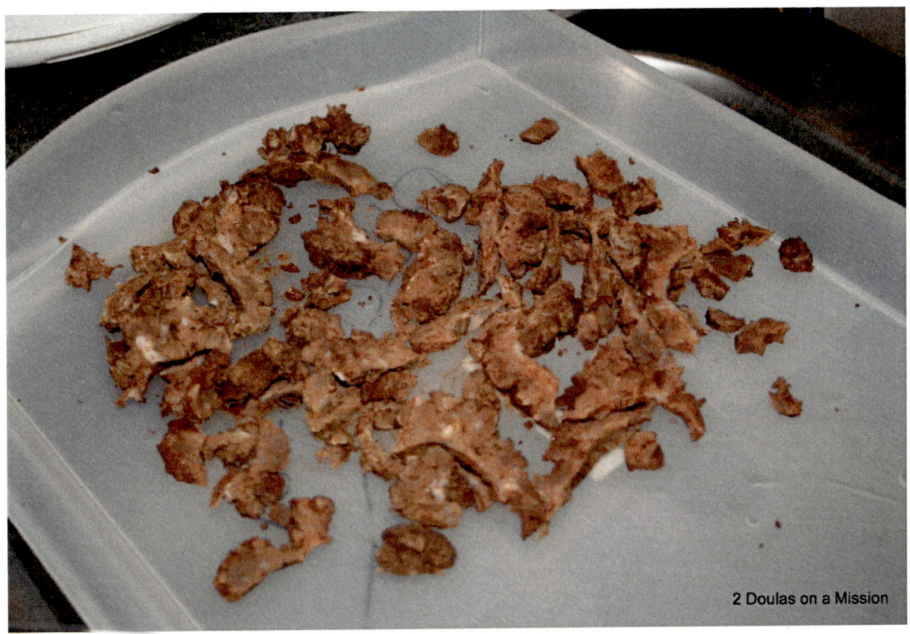

{placenta pieces steamed, cut and ready to be dehydrated}

- If using parchment paper, line your dehydrator trays now
- See the "Raw Method" for photos of the following steps
- Place the pieces in a single layer on your dehydrator trays
- Place the trays inside the dehydrator and set the temperature at 115 degrees. Typical drying time is 10-15 hours, sometimes longer, depending on how large/thick the placenta pieces are.
- If you don't have a dehydrator and are not concerned about temperature - you can lay the pieces of placenta out on a cookie sheet and dehydrate at the lowest temperature setting in your oven. Check every couple of hours.

- To determine if your placenta is done: remove several different pieces from the dehydrator to test. They should all snap in half with absolutely no moisture present.
- Once your pieces are dry, put them into your grinder. If you're using a coffee grinder it may take several rounds to get all of the pieces.
- Dump your powder onto your second tray
- Load capsule maker with the first round of empty capsules.
- Use the spreader card to scoop the powder into the capsule maker
- Use the tamper to tamp down once
- Use the spreader card to scoop some more powder into the capsules
- Use the spreader card to smooth everything out and remove excess powder
- Push the top part and the bottom part of the capsule maker together and voila – sealed capsules.
- Repeat until you have used all of your placenta powder

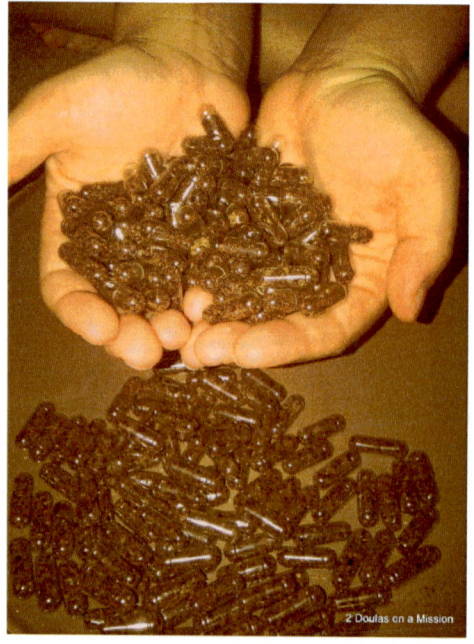

Dosage & Storage

I would by making it up if I told you a dosage – anyone would. Each placenta is different in size, weight and overall composition. Each woman's need is different. A general starting point would be 2 capsules 2 times per day. Some women take them with food, some don't. Some don't take them too late in the day as it gives them too much energy, others don't feel this at all. Dosage is completely self regulated and you'll just have to play around with it. If you have a specific goal in mind – a higher milk supply, less mood swings, etc. then take more. If you're having an especially bad day – maybe take a few more than you would on a good day. Once you find your sweet spot – stay there for a week or so and then gradually take a bit less and see what happens. The capsules are ideal for your immediate postpartum period and the goal is to gently wean yourself off of your placenta.

Keep your capsules in cool, dry place – a dark cupboard or even the refrigerator is ideal.

There are different schools of thought on how long your placenta is "good" for. The reality is – it never goes bad. It is fully dehydrated and thus, preserved. The potency of the placenta may be lower five years down the line, but this is true of any supplement, herb or vitamin.

Resources

Books:

Placenta: The Forgotten Chakra, by Robin Lim (http://gaia-d.com/robin-lim-e-books/)

Placenta: The Gift of Life, by Cornelia Enning (http://www.midwiferytoday.com/books/placenta.asp)

Articles:

The Amazing Placenta, by Sarah Buckley, M.D. (http://www.mothering.com/community/a/the-amazing-placenta)

The Amazing Placenta, by Suzanne Nguyen (http://m.theatlantic.com/health/archive/2013/12/the-amazing-placenta/282280/)

Check out our website for ways to connect with us via our social media outlets where we frequently post new articles and information on placenta love.

Made in the USA
San Bernardino, CA
04 December 2014